AF417888

Artificial Intelligence in Healthcare: possibilities and challenges

Anna Wohlthat

Impressum

Copyright: Anna Wohlthat
Jahr:

ISBN: 9789403613437

Lektorat/ Korrektorat: Anna Wohlthat
Illustrationen: Anna Wohlthat
Covergestaltung: Anna Wohlthat
Weitere Mitwirkende: kein

Verlagsportal: BS Business and Technology AG
Gedruckt in Deutschland

Die Deutsche Nationalbibliothek verzeichnet diese Publikation in der Deutschen Nationalbibliografie (falls zwei Pflichtexemplare an die DNB geschickt werden!).

Das Werk, einschließlich aller seiner Teile, ist urheberrechtlich geschützt. Jede Verwertung ist ohne Zustimmung des Verfassers unzulässig

Table of Content

1. Introduction

Artificial Intelligence has already entered the medical and biomedical fields; it works with data, could learn and collect experience. Many good practices are evidence that Artificial Intelligence became a useful tool in helping to diagnose and treat patients. Along with the undeniable advantages, there are a number of problems with its use in such an ethically sensitive area as medicine, as well as the issues of distribution of responsibility, job losses, and a number of concerns about an "uprising of robots" that is from fantastic spectrum.

The growing demand for clinical trials, treatment simulations, and new research are driving the rapid growth of Artificial Intelligence in healthcare.

1.1.   Goals and objectives of the study

The aim of this thesis is to analyze the factors and economic effect of Artificial Intelligence use at an orthopedic clinic, which specializes in outpatient treatment of patients.

The objectives of this study:

-        To outline the main problems that are associated with the introduction of AI into society in general and medical institutions in particular.

-        To define the basic concepts of Artificial Intelligence and consider the use of AI at the good practices in healthcare – medicine and economics.

-        To consider the main directions and the economic effect of the using AI in the activities of a medical institution at all levels (management, service, doctors, and patients).

-        To provide examples of the changes in the activities and business processes of a medical institution and the possible alterations of the economic changes after the introduction of a number of the AI-based technologies and applications.

-        To analyze and consider the prospects of AI application for the economic growth of the medical organization.

2. Artificial Intelligence: from chess player to neural networks

2.1. Artificial Intelligence: Stages of development

If we consider the historical plan for the creation and development of the AI, then the roots of the very idea of an intelligent machine go back to the 19th century, namely, to the idea of the mathematician Charles Babbage to create a chess machine capable of calculating moves. It was this idea that came to life more than 100 years later: in 1954, the American researcher William Whewell hired a group of analysts to write a chess program.

It was in the 50s of the last century that interest in Artificial Intelligence was extremely high, even bordering on sci-fiction. It was then that the term "Artificial Intelligence (AI)" appeared in the USA (in 1956). However, since computer technology was at the initial stage of development at that time, complex operations and calculations were practically impossible. In addition, the algorithms for the operation of a smart machine were themselves, more or less science fiction. This is why AI has frustrated scientists such a long time (Russel/Norvig 2016, p. 17).

The real boom of interest, research and patents related to AI began in the 1990s.

In 1997, the idea of chess intelligence was brought to life by IBM. Their development, Deep Blue, beats the world chess champion (Russel/Norvig 2016, p.29). New developments like IBM Watson and AlphaGo from Google followed. It was AlphaGo that became a breakthrough, since when playing Go, the player must be able to think creatively; the degree of abstraction is too great and there are too many scenarios for the development of events. In other words. when creating AlphaGo, it was proved that AI can not only count, but also can think.

This was followed by a poker tournament including AI, where it was demonstrated that it is able to understand when a player is bluffing. A computer can be trained from practice that if it has a weak hand and it bluffs, it can make additional money (cf. Hernandez 2019, p. n/a).

Over the past 10 years, AI has been used in many areas of our society.

First of all, thanks to the huge investments in its development made by technology giants (Facebook, Google, Amazon, Apple, Microsoft, etc.), AI is finding an ever wider application in many software products and technologies.

Nowadays, Artificial Intelligence is successfully used in advertising, marketing, trade, telecom, insurance, linguistics, banking and fintech.

2.2.   Artificial Intelligence. Definition

Artificial intelligence is "the ability of a digital computer or computer-controlled robot to perform tasks commonly associated with intelligent beings" (Copeland 2020, p. n/a).

Artificial Intelligence might be defined as computer science field that develops intelligent computer systems, i.e. systems that have capabilities, which we traditionally associate with the human mind - understanding language, learning, reasoning, problem solving, etc. (cf. Barr/Feigenbaum 1981, p. 3-4)

Jeff Bezos (CEO of Amazon) writes about Artificial Intelligence in the following way: "Over the past decades computers have broadly automated tasks programmers could describe with clear rules and algorithms. Modern Machine Learning techniques now allow us to do the same for tasks where describing the precise rules is much harder" (Banzhaf et al. 2020, p. 308).

Thus, we are talking about Artificial Intelligence when it comes to programs and machines that are able to independently make decisions and draw conclusions without having clear "rules of the game", analyzing gigantic data sets, comparing and drawing conclusions, and making decisions.

2.3.   Prediction, Big Data, learning and independent problem solving without clear rules

The most common uses of Artificial Intelligence are forecasting various scenarios and situations, assessing information and making conclusions based on such assessments, as well as searching for hidden patterns - data mining.

It is prediction that is the main difference between Artificial Intelligence and other computer software: when writing a program, a computer programmer knows at the initial stage what conclusion the machine should come, but with Artificial Intelligence, only the initial data is known. Artificial Intelligence makes comparisons and conclusions; it makes prediction and decisions, and is able to draw conclusions..

In order for Artificial Intelligence to make comparisons and conclusions, it certainly needs data. The more data, the greater accuracy can be achieved when obtaining a result. "AI will transform many industries. But it's not magic" (Ng 2016, p. n/a).

Big Data has become a breakthrough for the development of technologies based on AI. Researchers speak of "Big Data" as the main "raw material" of the 21st century (cf. Berners-Lee/Shadbolt 2011, p. n/a).

The term "Big Data" in the literature refers to all datasets that are too large or too complex to be estimated manually or using conventional electronic data processing tools. On closer inspection of the "Big Data" topic, one will quickly notice that this term is currently undergoing constant changes. As a rule, the area of "Big Data" is also associated with technologies that are required for collecting and analyzing data.

Continuously progressing digitalization takes place in almost all areas of life. As a consequence, there is an increasing amount of stored data. Experts even note a certain rhythm in this process: a doubling of existing data every two years (cf. Monnappa 2020, p. n/a).

Harry Shum (Microsoft AI and Research) highlights 3 main forces that made the dreams about Artificial Intelligence come true: increased computing power in the cloud, powerful algorithms that run on deep neural networks, and access to massive amounts of data (cf. Shum 2017, p. n/a).

McKinsey & Company in their research "Big Data – a revolution in the healthcare" include both issues related to the system of mutual settlements and the prevention of unnecessary treatment, as well as the issues related to the traditional methods of drug treatment. Finally, it is the identification of traditional structures affecting fee-for-payments and the issues of possible long-term cost recovery through the accumulated experience in the field of "Big Data" (cf. Groves et al. 2013, p. 10).

3. Basic concepts of AI

3.1. Neural networks and machine learning - the basic concepts of Artificial Intelligence

On a comparatively still short path of development of Artificial Intelligence, there was a search for the most successful algorithms and mathematical models for constructing Artificial Intelligence: 1. Linear regression; 2. Logistic regression; 3. Linear discriminant analysis; 4. Decision trees; 5. Naive Bayes; 6. K-Nearest Neighbors; 7. Learning vector quantization; 8. Support vector machines; 9. Bagging and random forest; 10. Deep neural networks (cf. Fedak 2018, p. n/a).

In real life, one comes across complex tasks that require serious studies and more complex solutions than the simplest machine learning algorithms. In such cases, neural networks come to the rescue.

A neural network is "a series of algorithms that seek to identify relationships in a data set via a process that mimics how the human brain works" (Chen 2020, p. n/a). The basic elements of neural networks are inputs (input values, most often two-dimensional arrays, where records are rows and features are columns), hidden layers (layers of the neural network in which the weights of each of the parameters are adjusted) and outputs (output values, most often probabilities belonging to different classes). The hidden layers consist of interconnected nodes, each of which is a perceptron (the simplest component of a neural network, an analogue of one neuron, which includes inputs; they are assigned different weights and subsequently the weights are changed to approximate the desired classification's result) (Chen 2020, p. n/a).

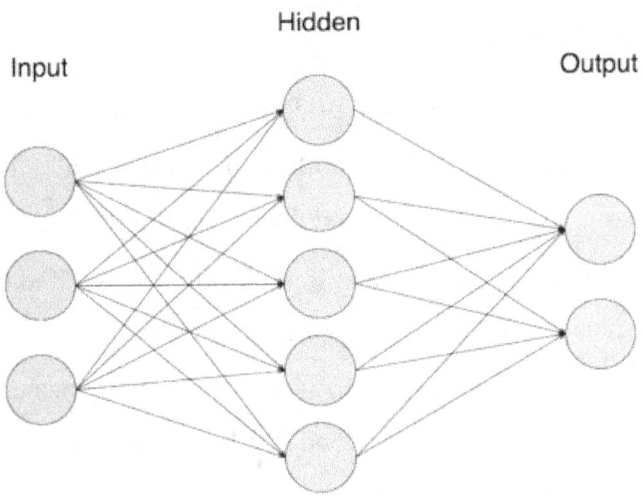

Figure 1. The structure of the neural network. (Dacombe, 2017).

Currently, there are many models for the implementation of neural networks. There are "classic" single-layer neural networks that are used to solve simple problems.

There are mathematical models in which the output of one neural network is directed to the input of another; in this way, cascades of connections are created, the so-called multilayer neural networks (MNN) and one of their most powerful options - convolutional neural network (CNN). MNNs have great computing power, but they also require huge computing resources.

Recurrent neural networks (RNNs) are another type of neural networks. We speak of these networks when the output from the network layer is transmitted back as a feedback to one of the inputs. Such platforms have a "memory effect", and they are able to track the dynamics of changes in input factors.

Machine learning (ML) is an application of Artificial Intelligence that provides systems with the ability to automatically learn and improve from experience without being explicitly programmed. Machine learning focuses on the development of computer programs that can access data and use it to learn for themselves (Bohr/Memarzadeh 2020, p.68). Machine learning assumes that instead of creating programs manually by using a special set of instructions to perform a specific task - a machine can be trained by using a large amount of data and algorithms. The data and algorithms will enable it to learn how to perform a task on its own or with the help of a so-called "teacher" (examples, training data).

ML is a complex process of finding patterns in data and making predictions based on them. Machine Learning uses algorithms that enable a computer to make inferences from available data. Arthur Samuel created the term Machine Learning in 1959 while he was at IBM. A fashionable description of machine learning is due to Samuel, who called the machine learning an area of the computer science that provides computers the capability to learn without being explicity automated. (Dasgupta 2018, p. 219)

3.2. Types of Machine Learning

There are 3 types of ML: Supervised learning, Reinforcement learning, and Unsupervised learning (cf. Russel/Norvig 2016, p. 695).

One more type Semisupervised learning is also considered by some researchers as a separate type of ML, although it is a mix between Supervised and Unsupervised types (Bohr/Memarzadeh 2020, p.70).

<u>Supervised learning:</u>

In supervised learning, specially selected data is used, in which the correct answers are already known and reliably determined, and the parameters of the neural network are adjusted so as to minimize errors. In this way, AI can match the correct answers to each input example and identify possible dependencies of the answer on the input data. For example, a collection of X-ray images with the indicated conclusions will be the basis for teaching AI, i.e., they will be its "teacher". From a series of obtained models, a person eventually chooses the most suitable one, for example, according to the maximum accuracy of the forecasts that are issued.

In this method, there are a number of risks: the subjectivity of the person who selects the data, the limitation of the conceptual model resulting from the current level of scientific development, which creates a "blindness" to AI. Prediction can be unpredictable and affects the accuracy of the mathematical mode negatively (cf. Russel/Norvig 2016, p. 695-697).

Reinforcement learning

AI learns on the base of interaction with the environmental world, it generates pairs (factor-right answer) and itself learns from them through the system of rewards and punishments (cf. Russel/Norvig 2016, p. 695).

Unsupervised learning

Unsupervised learning is used where there are no pre-prepared answers and classification algorithms. In this case, the AI focuses on the independent identification of hidden dependencies and the search for ontology (cf. Gusev/Dobridnyuk 2017, p. 90).

No labels are given to the learning algorithm, leaving it on its own to find structure in its input. It is used for clustering population in different groups. Unsupervised learning can be a goal in itself (discovering hidden patterns in data) (cf. Russel/Norvig 2016, p. 694).

Nowadays, neural networks cope with many tasks much better than humans. For example, there are neural networks that determine what is shown on a photograph with much greater accuracy than humans. However, there are ways to "crash" almost any neural network of this type, and make mistakes in determining what is shown on the photo.

For example, AI can detect the image of an elephant completely infallibly in standard conditions and situations, but AI cannot detect an elephant if it is placed in a room on a sofa. The situation is too unrealistic and not typical. But a child 2-3 years old will immediately and infallibly determine that an elephant is sitting on the sofa (cf. Rosenfeld et al. 2018, p.2-3).

Deep Learning methods of neural networks are used to solve many data processing problems (cf. Lee et al. 2018, p. 112).

Supervised learning is preferable when there is a large amount of reliable data. In cases where databases with mapped information are lacking or insufficient, self-learning based on Deep Learning should be applied. Such decisions do not require expert supervision.

3.3. Deep learning and neural networks for complex solutions. BlackBox problem

Recently, it is neural networks, in combination with deep learning that have been accepted as the most popular technological solutions in the field of AI.

The science that studies deep neural networks is called Deep Learning. At the moment, this area is developing rapidly, thanks to its unsurpassed usefulness to society.

It is not difficult to understand how a perceptron or the simplest neural network of several neurons is designed. However, the large neural networks with a huge number of layers (for example, the newest neural network EfficientNet B7 has 813 layers (cf. Stiedemann 2020, p. n/a) are a mystery to humans in terms of internal mechanics. This concept is called the Black Box Problem (cf. O'Neil 2016, p.18).

Imagine a situation: a new algorithm is used to determine the suspect risk of any disease. We provide demographic data about a person, his/her personal information, and previous health problems. Then, we see some kind of result, for example, a high risk of diabetes. What is this conclusion based on? Yes, we used some data to train this model, but how much weight has each characteristic received? Thus, for example, if our training sample has more people with any particular social status or life-style, the model will give a lot of weight to this characteristic and will be subject to human prejudice (cf. Bohr/ Memarzadeh 2020, p.490).

Now, many companies are busy creating so-called Explainable Artificial Intelligence, new machine learning models that can explain how classification is made, which parameters prevail in importance and how the algorithm works in general (cf. Arrieta et al. 2020, p. n/a).

3.4. Solving problems of varying complexity. Use of the Linear regression, Logit, Random Forest methods

When choosing the most appropriate machine learning algorithm, it is important to look at the scale of the problem and its characteristics. Often people who are poorly versed in machine learning are perplexed, about why fairly simple algorithms are used for tasks, such as Linear regression, Logit, and Random Forest, when there are various neural networks that have state-of-the-art accuracy?

However, simple problems require simple solutions. It is important to objectively assess the problem before selecting the appropriate algorithm.

Let us imagine a physical experiment in which we determine the dependence of temperature on pressure. We run an experiment and write the values into a table. Then, we build a linear regression in order to estimate the dependence of these values.

Of course, we could have used an advanced regression model (a type of supervised learning), for example, ElasticNet Regression, but most likely the result would be the same, but much more computer power and time would be spent.

Clustering is another example of the aforementioned problem. There are many techniques for this type of unsupervised learning. However, most often the simplest K-Means algorithm is used for clustering several variables. In it, even the use of the more complex distance metrics (an equation that describes how far the points should be from the center of the cluster) gives undesirable results. Let's say we would like to categorize shopping mall's shoppers into clusters for targeting advertising funds (discounts, thank you letters, surveys about desired products) based on their annual income and spending level in the mall. If we use the K-means clustering with Euclidian distance metric (the simplest version of the metric), then we will get good results that meet our expectations.

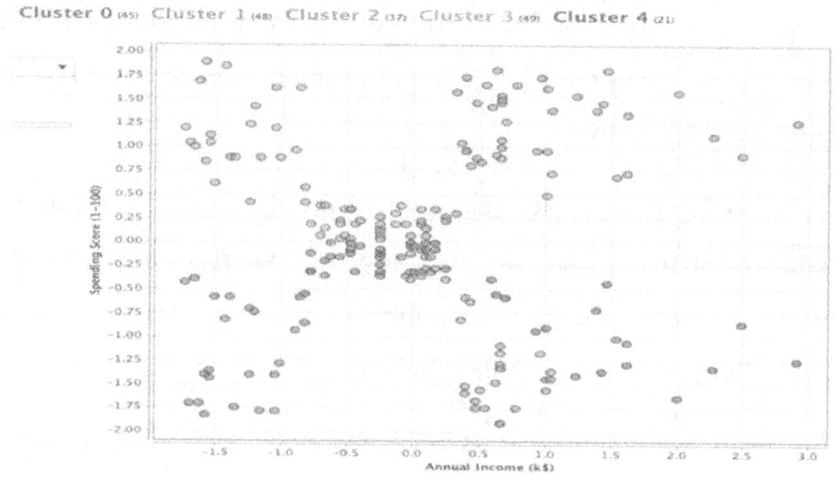

Figure 2. Scatter plot of points in 5 clusters. Euclidian distance metric.

(Own illustration)

Using a more complex distance metric, we get completely incomprehensible clusters that will not help us in targeting promotions.

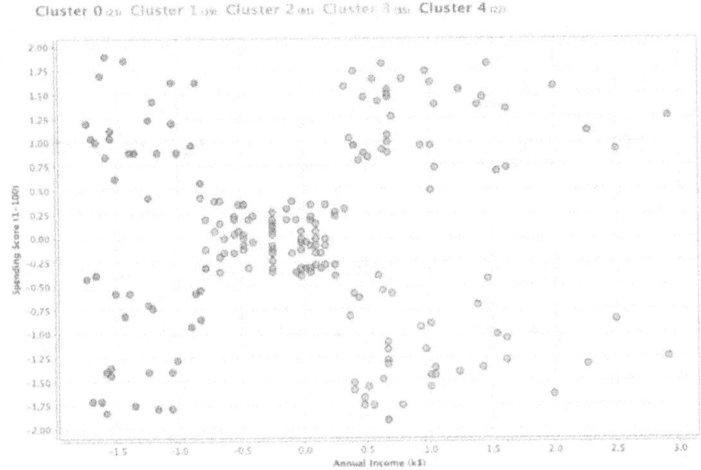

Figure 3. Scatter plot of points in 5 clusters. Cosine similarity distance metric.

(Own illustration)

Thus, the simple tasks require classical simple machine learning algorithms, since this gives good results and at the same time is efficient in terms of the consumption of computer power and time.

4. Artificial Intelligence's ecosystem in medicine

4.1. Artificial Intelligence market

Artificial Intelligence market consists of many companies and institutions that perform their specific tasks and functions. Although the modern ecosystem in this market as a whole is still being formed, one can already imagine what its shape will be in the near future.

One way to classify the players in the following market is suggested by SafeGraph CEO Auren Hoffman, who catogorizes the machine learning and AI companies into three types: Superrich; Servicers; Innovators (cf. Hoffman 2016, p. n/a). This division strongly resembles the paradigm of other, more classical markets.

Companies of the Superrich type are AI companies with their own data. These are companies such as Google, Facebook, Baidu, Tencent, Amazon, Microsoft and others. There are not many of such companies in the world, but they have a significant advantage: since they have access to huge reservoirs of purified and structured data, the engineers of these companies can develop AI technologies based on the resources available, and they can further develop their algorithms and approaches (cf. Hoffman 2016, p. n/a).

Servicer companies help other companies process massive amounts of data. They can process huge clusters of data, including unstructured data, and add the necessary insights. These companies are service companies, because they do not have their own data, but they work with the data of their customers. One of these successful companies is Palantir Technologies, which is a very popular solution in the US government, and it helps them understand data with minimal costs. Other examples are IBM, HP, and Oracle, as well as various consulting companies and oter companies that provide solutions to help large corporations improve some aspect of their business, for example, pricing, logistics, or customer service (cf. Hoffman 2016, p. n/a).

The innovation company-type focuses on solving a specific problem, but does not have its own data and does not provide services to other companies. Examples of such companies are Two Sigma Investments and Point72 Asset Management, which spend millions of dollars on data because they do not generate the data themselves. Other examples are Cruise Automation, which focuses on the development of self-driving cars and it was recently acquired by GM and Flatiron Health, which is engaged in cancer research. After acquiring data, such companies also have to clean it, merge it, i.e. carry out preliminary ETL procedures before starting to work with it (cf. Hoffman 2016, p. n/a).

Superrich companies have powerful advantages over the rest. However, it can be assumed that as data access becomes more democratic, companies from the other two groups will nevertheless grow at a high rate. An example of this democratization is Yahoo, which posted 13.5 TB of data on how users behaved on the Yahoo homepage and on the pages of individual services of the company. Another example is Criteo, a developer of technology solutions for advertising, which published 1 TB of data.

According to IDC experts, companies such as Amazon, Alphabet, IBM and Microsoft will own 60% of AI platforms. These companies now also dominate in the cloud computing business. At the same time, each company mentioned, when taken separately, is building its own ecosystem (cf. Ostrovskiy 2017, p. n/a)

4.2. Artificial Intelligence in medicine

Artificial Intelligence in medicine is one of the most promising, but at the same time, one of the most difficult spheres of social life. Including the introduction of AI here is bound to face certain obstacles.

Medicine is one of the industries that has many prospects for the introduction of both machine learning, natural language processing, as well as robotics.

Up to date, there have been a large number of successful cases involving the application of AI in medicine and healthcare.

One can distinguish between 4 main areas of AI services:

- Diagnostics

- Automatization of doctors' work, including robotization

- Selection of treatment methods

- Biopharmaceuticals

In medicine, one can talk about an existing contradiction. On the one hand, it is one of the most rapidly and actively developing branches of scientific knowledge: many scientists are engaged in the development of new methods of both diagnosis and treatment. In general, biopharmaceuticals is an industry in which huge investments are made. However, on the other hand, the medical field is perhaps the most undemocratic and stagnant industry in terms of providing information, as well as the doctor-patient relationship.

Physicians continue to view the patients in today's digital world as objects rather than equal partners. There is a perception that medicine will not be able to move forward if consumers continue to be suppressed or treated as second-class people. In medicine, paternalism dominates - a decisive force that does not allow moving forward. It will require not only a change in culture within the medical community, but also new technologies that stimulate the process from the outside (cf. Bohr/Memarzadeh 2020, p. 49-51).

The latest technical means make it easy to accomplish what seemed impossible yesterday, simplifying the lives of doctors and patients.

The development of technology and the massive consumer access to smart gadgets are completely changing the balance of power, opportunities and order of relationships in medicine. Machine learning technologies significantly speed up the doctor's work and improve the quality of his/her work.

The medicine of the future is not based on one technology or device. It is a whole ecosystem, based on the prevention of diseases - a healthy diet, a healthy lifestyle, early diagnosis and, if necessary, minimally invasive treatment that is followed by home rehabilitation (cf. Kuznetzov 2018, p. n/a).

Artificial Intelligence, as it exists in medicine is used fairly widely, and it is used both in clinical practice and in the auxiliary processes of a medical organization.

4.3. The use of Artificial Intelligence in clinical practice. Good practices

The introduction of the Artificial Intelligence-based programs and the development of technologies in general have facilitated the use of AI in medicine.

Today, AI's developers have managed to address a range of deficiencies in healthcare with AI and they have developed applications and solutions to improve both productivity and quality of care in healthcare practices and clinics by providing exceptional ease of use (cf. De 2017, p. n/a).

In accordance with the Allied Market Research report, "The AI in healthcare market was valued at $4,836.87million in 2019 and is projected to reach $99,491.58 million by 2027, registering a CAGR of 42.8% from 2020 to 2027" (Joshi/Sumant 2020, p. n/a) .

The use of AI in medicine pursues, first of all, the reduction of health care costs and the corresponding need to limit them.

Another motivation is the problem of the quality of diagnostics: circa 20-30% of medical research is either inaccurate or interpreted inaccurately. Thus, there is a desire to standardize and automate the routine functions up to the creation of self-guided diagnostic models (cf. Morozov 2018, p. n/a).

4.4. Areas of Artificial Intelligence's application in medicine

4.4.1. Artificial Intelligence for diagnostic

Artificial Intelligence can be used for diagnosis. AI, based on a patient's data and image analysis, is able to make a diagnosis. The use of Artificial Intelligence can massively improve diagnostic accuracy.

The most popular, largest, and most talked about use of AI in diagnostics is the IBM Watson cognitive system (www.ibm.com/watson-health). In order to train AI of the IBM Watson, 30 billion medical images were analyzed, for which IBM had to buy Merge Healthcare for $ 1 billion. The system was originally planned for the diagnosis of cancer, but the capabilities of IBM Watson were expanded. At this stage, Watson Artificial Intelligence interprets text and images, acts as a radiologist assistant, assists cardiologists in diagnosing and finding signs of heart valve stenosis, and analyzes ultrasound images, X-rays and other graphical information in order to clarify the diagnosis. In addition to the heart problems, Watson is able to refine the diagnosis of cancer patients, diagnose patients with pulmonary diseases or brain problems by using medical images and additional information. In the near future, the developers plan to further expand the capabilities of Watson, directing its ability to diagnose deep vein thrombosis, cardiomyopathy, and various types of heart attacks (cf. Topol 2019, loc.953).

Watson asks questions and makes guesses by using the latest medical research in oncology along with information from the patient's medical record and current symptoms. As a result, each patient receives an individual approach. After all, the same disease, even in its simplest and most harmless forms, progresses differently in different people.

The system is capable of analyzing huge amounts of data, and this is unstructured data, where the system systematizes everything and makes objective conclusions.

IBM Watson offers each patient a personalized course of treatment, which is aimed at those factors that led to the development of the disease by taking into account each patient's genome. This increases the chances of a successful recovery, and each new case increases this likelihood even more (cf. Agadzhanov 2015, p. n/a).

At the same time, Watson studies the latest data on a specific disease or a group of diseases - an ordinary doctor simply cannot study all the necessary information. At best, we are talking about several thematic articles based on research results. IBM Watson, on the other hand, can structure huge amounts of data in seconds, while simultaneously studying the results of research on a specific topic over the past couple of years.

The advantages of the system are that it is capable of processing huge amounts of data in a very short period, which no doctor or group of doctors is able to do.

In addition, the system solves the issue of highly qualified medical personnel.

Problems with Watson are completely correlated with health problems in general. These are problems in interoperability (interaction of different systems with each other) and data collection. For example, there is a discrepancy in the maintenance of medical records. Thus, a problem with their management arises. That is why it turned out that teaching a computer to work in real conditions in the healthcare system turned out to be much more difficult than planned (cf. Ross/Swetlitz 2017, p. n/a).

Another concern stems from the fact that Watson's primary source of diagnostic information is a group of experts from Memorial Sloan Kettering Cancer Center (USA). Although the hospital is considered one of the best cancer centers in the world, experts believe this approach, leads to Watson producing biased results that can only be applied to wealthy patients (cf. Topol 2019, loc.974).

The issue of AI bias is of great concern, especially given the differences in data that exist for certain populations, for example, minorities or bi-sexual people. Another group of experts notes that companies like IBM which want to capitalize on AI in healthcare must first address the issue of data availability in this industry (cf. Ross/Swetlitz 2017, p. n/a).

One can say that Watson, like any innovative product, did not set explicit economic goals for its creators. The development cost of its components were usually higher than planned, and its content was quite cumbersome when compared with traditional healthcare budgets. That is why several hospitals that took part in initial tests withdrew from the project (cf. Ross/Swetlitz 2017, p. n/a). Even today, it can be considered as an experimental testing ground. Tested prototypes can be transferred to serial production, achieving higher performance in terms of price-quality criterion and suitability for service in real conditions (cf. Gusev/Dobridnyuk 2017, p. 90).

Watson is a versatile system. However, there are also many specialized systems that focus on a single disease. The largest number of AI's developments are in the field of diagnosis and treatment of cancer.

The IBM Watson ecosystem is now home to tens of thousands of developers, entrepreneurs and other enthusiasts who have built thousands of applications using Watson Zone on Bluemix, which is IBM's Platform as a Service (PaaS) solution. Bluemix allows anyone to use 100 tools, which include Watson services, to efficiently create, run and manage applications in any cloud environment (Ostrovskiy 2017, p. 7).

Another example is Freenome (www.freenome.com). It aims at an early diagnosis of disease susceptibility.

The Freenome multiomics platform detects key biological signals based on a blood test. The platform combines DNA, methylation and protein analysis with advanced computational biology and machine learning techniques for early cancer detection. There is a large number of developments in the field of diagnostics of various diseases.

Most often, similar diagnostics by using AI is aimed at the diagnosis and prognosis of oncological and dermatology diseases, and improving diabetes prediction. All applications are based on the analysis of genomic factors or images. It includes conventional (for the diagnosis of melanoma, for example) and MRI / X-ray images (neurology, diseases of the musculoskeletal system, oncology, etc.)

The Israeli company MaxQ-AI (www.maxq.ai) has developed a solution based on AI and Big Data, thanks to which doctors can more accurately diagnose a stroke. In order to do this, in real time, the MedyMatch system compares the image of the patient's brain with hundreds of thousands of other images that are in its "cloud". It is known that strokes can be caused by two reasons: cerebral hemorrhage and blood clot. Accordingly, each of these cases requires a different approach to treatment. However, according to statistics, despite improvements in CT, the number of errors in diagnosis has not changed over the past 30 years. At approximately 30% it means that in almost every third case, the doctor prescribes the wrong treatment for the patient, which often leads toregretful consequences. The MedyMatch system is able to track the smallest deviations from the norm that a specialist can not always notice. As a result, this minimizes the likelihood of errors in diagnosing and prescribing a treatment.

4.4.2. Telemedicine

Telemedicine or AI-based programs that provide the conditions of a "home hospital". Patients have to be constantly aware of their own health status. Wearables, which allow them to monitor pulse, pressure, breathing and other health indicatorsare of great assistance in this. According to the information received, it is necessary to do something at the moment (take medicine, change the type of physical activity, etc.

One of the most proven and "capable" applications combining telemedicine with chat bot in medicine today is the German ADA Health system. The system has existed for nine years and is continuously being improved. It currently has about 10 million users, and supports 7 languages, including the rare Kiswahili (Tanzania). ADA (https://ada.com) is a company founded by doctors, programmers, scientists, creating new opportunities for maintaining personal health. The application is very easy to use.

The ADA chatbot asks the consumer a range of questions related to his/her complaints. During the interview, the patient is given explanations of certain terms about which the question is asked. After a series of questions (circa 30), a presumptive diagnosis is issued based on an assessment of the patient's answers. Then, it reports the likelihood of a particular disease, while giving detailed explanations which of the named symptoms influenced the system conclusions. If necessary, the application connects the patient with a real doctor in chat for a consultation.

Another example of a telemedicine chatbot is the English Babylon (https://www.babylonhealth.com). This chatbot app even partners with the National Health Service of England (NHS) (cf. Nunez 2017, p. n/a) as the first line for patients seeking medical attention. Babylon also offers online consultation with a doctor. The main directions of treatment are the most frequent complaints with which patients go to the ambulance: food poisoning, fever, abdominal pain, or impetigo. During the COVID-19 pandemic, the app helps patients check their symptoms and guide them in their next steps.

Despite the presence of a number of successful applications, a certain amount of time should pass before the widespread implementation of telemedicine chatbots that diagnose patients by themselves. Currently, the bots can collect information and give advice, thereby reducing the likelihood of errors and saving the time of the doctors and patients.

4.4.3. Biomedical research

Artificial Intelligence searches for new or the most effective molecules for drugs. There, AI can study, predict and interpret how genetic variations change important cellular processes and lead to disease. Thus, the knowledge of the cause of the disease can make therapy more efficient)

4.4.4. Analysis and prediction

Systems of analysis and prediction of events are also tasks that Artificial Intelligence can solve nowadays and where they can have a significant effect. For example, the operational analysis of the incidence of the changes can quickly predict a change in patient attendance at health care organizations or the need for medications.

Harvard University's teaching hospital, Beth Israel Deaconess Medical Center uses AI to diagnose potentially deadly blood diseases at a very early stage. They have developed and use a microscope, enhanced by AI that might help clinical microbiologists diagnose potentially deadly blood infections and improve patients' odds for survival (cf. Mitchell 2017, p. n/a).

4.4.5. Robotics and mechatronics

Development of robotics and mechatronics. The well-known robotic surgeon DaVinci is only the first step towards, replacing doctors with machines, or at the least towards improving the quality of work of the medical staff. The integration of robotics with AI is now seen as one of the most promising areas, thanks to which it will be possible to shift routine operations to machines, including in medicine.

4.5. Application of Artificial Intelligence in the management of medical institutions. Good practices.

•	Speech recognition and natural language understanding systems – chatbots used to register patients, answer questions asked at the call center level, call patients with reminders about appointments, collecting opinions, etc. Automated patient's support chatbots can be of great help in promoting healthy lifestyles and adherence to treatment. Chatbots can already learn to answer routine questions, suggest the tactics of patient behavior in simple situations, connect the patient with the right doctor by telecommunication devices, give dietary recommendations, etc. Such a development of healthcare towards self-service and greater involvement of patients in maintaining their health without a visit to the doctor can save significant financial resources.

•	Systems for automatic classification and verification of information (Digital Patient's History) can help to link patient information in various forms and in various information systems. For example, it will be possible to build an integral electronic medical record from individual episodes, described in differing degrees of detail, without clear or contradictory structuring of information. Such digitization can facilitate the work of physicians. Moreover, it will also have economic benefits for the entire healthcare system, because the cost of unnecessary examinations, tests, analyses, etc. will be reduced.

- Automatization of business processes and marketing solutions, including AI use in HR, accounting (Virtual assistants), marketing, advertising, etc.

A promising technology is the machine analysis of the content of social networks and Internet portals in order to quickly obtain sociological, demographic, or marketing information about the quality of the health care system and medical institutions for monitoring of reputation and public opinion about services. For example, using AI-based applications can be used for constant monitoring of comments appearing on the network and to work with objections.

4.5.1. Recommendation System

One of the most significant early marketing applications of AI was the Recommendation System on Amazon, which was launched in 1998. The recommendations were user-based. The algorithm searched for other users with similar interests to those of a particular user and it made recommendations for viewing certain products that others had already viewed, but the aforementioned user had not (cf. Smith/Linden 2017, p. n/a).

Such a system naturally had its drawbacks. It did not work exactly as planned, because every person is different, and finding similar people in real time is difficult due to the limited resources of online computing. However, Amazon's recommendation system has led to other similar systems on Netflix or Youtube.

Since then, platforms allowing content creation without the help of journalists or writers have been launched. The first such platform was Yahoo's Automated Insights Wordsmith platform. Such tools have significantly reduced the cost of content creation and made it possible to write targeted content separately for each user.

The changes have also affected advertising campaigns. In 2014, the first algorithms that optimized budget allocation between different advertising channels or keywords appeared. Such scripts also made it possible to automate the process of creating the advertising campaigns settings.

The year 2015 brought another sophisticated machine learning algorithm to humanity. RankBrain can analyze a series of user queries in Google search and return those links or products that the user most likely needs, based on his/her queries.

Interest in Artificial Intelligence has grown the fastest in recent years. Large companies and small businesses are adopting various Artificial Intelligence algorithms to increase profitability and to automate various processes. Social media and online shopping are using smart chatbots to reduce call center maintenance costs. More and more companies are collecting user data for targeted advertising. This is why the phenomenon of AI in marketing is promising and relevant.

The classical and the most common options for using AI in marketing are the following: a budget optimization for various advertising campaigns,choosing the most suitable keywords and parameters of advertising campaigns depending on various factors; drawing up a portrait of a buyer based on collecting data from Internet resources and analyzing his/her needs.

One of the most significant advances in Artificial Intelligence marketing is the personalization of content and ads. Previously, marketers had to develop an approach to each client by their means, but now AI's algorithms are able to develop an approach to any consumer, based on a set of data from the user's activity in the network and demographic data.

Internet contains a colossal amount of data about all of its users. Some of them:

- Information on social networks: age, gender, marital status.

-"Traces" on the Internet: likes, reposting, group memberships, friends lists, transitions on the websites.

- Cookie files, trackers on the websites

- Websites of organizations, clubs, universities, schools and other places where a person can work or study.

Thus, it is not difficult to analyze this data and collect hundreds or even thousands of different facts characterizing a person. With this amount of data, a well-trained neural network can quickly identify a potential buyer and show him/her an appropriate ad. For example, if a neural network receives a 19-year-old girl at an entry who is fond of dancing, then it is unlikely that she will be shown an advertisement for fishing rods. Most likely, she will see an advertisement for a new dance club in her city (also an important detail, since the location is one of leading ad targeting parameters).

Also, in addition to the demographic data, an analysis of the visits to the websites for a certain amount of time is widely used. For example, if a person looked at wedding dresses and a restaurant for a banquet, then most likely a wedding isplanned, and this person can be offered an advertisement for a wedding bouquet.

Let's take a look at how targeted advertising works from the inside. After receiving responses from various users about certain ads and placing them in a matrix, the algorithm programmatically creates the input data: custom matrices and ad matrices.

In the nodes of the matrix the linear representation of the features' values that reflect some users and ad's metrics also indicate a person's preference or ad characteristics. For such an action, one can use the LightFM library for Python, which acts as a "factorization machine and learning linear embeddings for each feature" (cf. Rival 2018, p. n/a).

After these steps, the library creates a new matrix (which is the product of the multiplication of two composite matrices) containing predicted scores for all ads and all users, so that even if the person has not yet estimated their expectations, we can see their expected reaction. Thus, by sorting the predicted reaction, we can show a user the most effective ad. This method is called linear factorization. This method is quite useful in terms of accuracy and power consumption of the computer. However, neural networks can be more accurate when dealing with the targeted ads.

The TensorRec library can be used to train a neural network, which is used to recommend ads to users. Instead of just the user's ratings, it also uses metadata about each user (age, gender, marital status) and ads (genre of the advertised movie, price). The result of the neural network is the score. The higher it is, the more likely the ad will be liked by a specific user. Such a neural network is presented as a classical neural network for classification – it compares the obtained scores and the user's real assessment: he or she likes it or does not like.

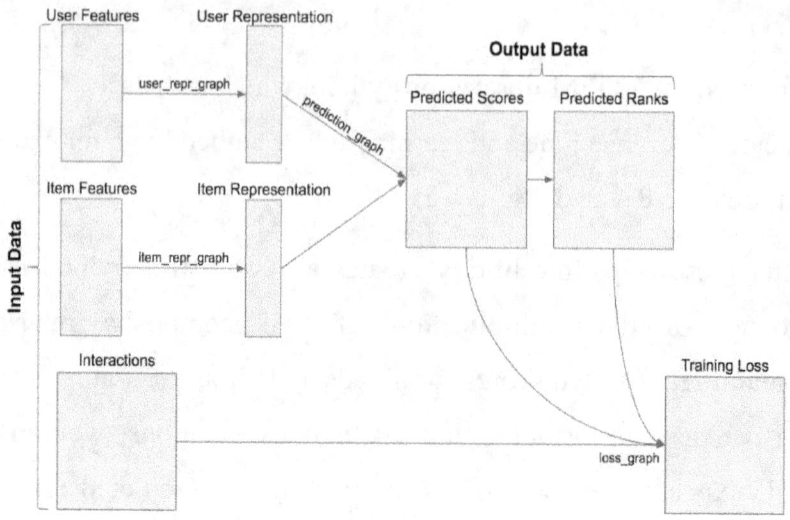

Figure 4: Recommendation System Neural Network Basic
Representation (Kirk 2017)

One example of the user's portrait recognition algorithms is
XANT (https://www2.xant.ai), a tool for marketers that, among
other useful features, provides practical help about each user. For
example, whether they would prefer to communicate via the
phone, or if a marketer should write to them via email. This
algorithm will immediately respond if the users are friendly and if
it is likely that an agreement can be reached with them. All of
these useful aspects of the customers' relationships are presented
in this program.

Artificial Intelligence algorithms on Internet collect a huge
amount of the user data in order to target ads as efficiently as
possible. From an ethical point of view, this issue is a sensitive
topic. Many websites and social networks prohibit parsing. For
example, Facebook can prosecute people who launch bots that

receive personal information from a social network. However, many sites such as Twitter allow bots to parse without any restrictions. Personalized advertising is firmly entrenched in people's lives, and continues to grow rapidly.

4.5.2. Artificial Intelligencen in marketing and advertising

In marketing and advertising it is also important to consider mechanisms for predicting future customer desires. These are based on the study of the user's previous activities.

The search engine starts searching for almost any product. Search engine algorithms allow real-time analysis of the user's request and give him/her the most relevant answers. These are some of the most important Artificial Intelligence applications for marketing.

An excellent example of such an algorithm is Google's RankBrain system. It is a self-learning Artificial Intelligence algorithm, built on various types of machine learning: supervised learning to learn elements of good search responses, unsupervised learning to cluster search results by topic. RankBrain itself improves the algorithm depending on the search query: it ranks by importance, novelty, by content, and by the user's previous search.

A question immediately arises: how does the algorithm understand our request more accurately than all previous technological solutions, and how is user's satisfaction assessed?

Firstly, RankBrain has introduced a new logic to searching for links to unfamiliar words: now the search does not take place on all Internet pages according to the appearance of keywords, but is instead based on previous search queries where these keywords appeared. This is partly due to Word2vec technology (a popular language analysis and word clustering technique), which turns words into concepts by vectorizing them.

Secondly, to understand the user's reaction to search results, several vital parameters are used: CTR (click-through rate), time spent on the site, pogo-sticking (a phenomenon when a user visits several sites from the search results in a short amount of time in order to find the most suitable result). The last concept is the most relevant for evaluating the effectiveness of the algorithm, since if the user immediately left the opened site, then, most likely, he/she is unhappy with it.

In this way, RankBrain helps advertisers to make sure that their ads are shown only when they are needed.

Another aspect of past action recommendations is retargeting (when ads appear on ads and social media with products that a user has recently viewed on another site). Retargeting is carried out using cookie files, i.e., a website using cookies follows the user and reminds of a product even on other sites through advertising. This mechanism is not entirely related to the machine learning, but it reflects how an algorithm can help sell a product that the user may have forgotten about by showing it to him/her many times.

Artificial Intelligence is capable not of only creating creative content, but also managing a company's budget by making ad purchases.

Optimizing the ad budget using a variety of mathematical tools is one powerful tool that can assist a marketer. Facebook was the first to provide this opportunity to the advertisers who place ads on their platform.

Thanks to AI, the marketer no longer needs to monitor the progress of advertising campaigns around the clock in order to optimize them. A smart algorithm does everything for him/her. In addition to the budget, there is a bid strategy in the budget optimization settings: a parameter that determines the tactics of the tool. More specifically, whether it will find the most profitable options and whether it will use them to the detriment of the rest, or it will leave approximately the same budget for each ad.

An algorithm for analyzing time intervals ARIMA or a neural network, for example, can make predictions about the effectiveness of individual advertisements, based on real-time data, such as target audience, time of the day, time of the year, or political sentiment. After that, the algorithm gives a conditional rating to all possible advertising campaigns in order to properly allocate the budget specifically for effective campaigns. After that, a mathematical optimization algorithm is put into action, which, by using the conditional rating of a specific ad, composes equations - one for the budget, the second for the total number of clicks or responses from the audience - and it optimizes the variables in them in such a way as to maximize the responses when fulfilling the budget.

From the point of view of mathematical optimization, the function is to maximize profit (clicks or reach), the variable is a priority in the advertising process, and the limitation is what budget must be within the specified parameters.

Another important part of this process is finding the most effective ads to display. According to Facebook itself, their dynamic ad system strives to show as many ads as possible within a budget. Since ads are placed on different platforms, it may turn out that due to the significant price difference between them, the ad will not reach the desired platform. Using simple components of the budget optimization engine, this is an innovative and convenient tool for advertisers.

4.5.3. Albert platform

All of the aforementioned processes are performed by various services to help marketers.

One of the most popular services for this is the Albert platform (www.albert.ai), which uses Artificial Intelligence algorithms to automate media purchases and the target settings. The service's clients include brands such as Harley-Davidson, Gallery Furniture, Natori, Dole Asia and others. According to the service, the platform can increase sales up to 87% and ROAS (return on investment in advertising) up to 517%. AI marketing has a great potential to improve ad performance while reducing its cost.

Albert, for example, completely takes over the management of advertising campaigns: from bidding and integration to distributing messages through different platforms (email, search engines and social networks). At the same time, "it" works faster than any specialist, and it can also determine various niches and patterns of shopping (cf. Wegert 2016, p. n/a). The downside is that Albert is only supported in English and it is also geared towards serving large companies with solid advertising budgets.

4.5.4. Origami platform

Another product with multilingual support is Origami (www.origami.ru). In addition to having multilingual support, this Artificial Intelligence is seen as a more budget option for small companies.

Origami - includes the following features:

- End-to-end performance analytics for advertising platforms (Yandex.Direct and Google Ads), with the integration of various statistics sources (Account Connection + Web

Analytics + Call Tracking + CRM). As a result, it details a campaign / phrase / group from click to order / income.

- Bid manager for Yandex.Direct. Retention strategies to reach / position in search results. A simple and reliable tool that is great for brand queries, for example, managing small accounts, where manual adjustments are not yet problematic. Places bids every 15-30-60 minutes. One can customize a strategy at the campaign level and at the phrase level.

- Automated rules in Direct and Ads (managing bids in the RK) for all advertising campaigns. One can customize different campaign's management logics. The "if – then" principle works at the campaign / phrase / site level for various metrics. The conditions under which the advertising campaigns work can be configured. For example, if there is an expense over X rubles and less than Y conversions in the campaign over the last seven days, then one changes the rate.

- Conversion Optimizer, which gives + 15-30% to the number of conversions or income in the first months of work. Conversion Optimizer - assigns bids automatically by focusing on statistics for phrases from web analytics, CRM, call tracking. The optimizer reallocates the budget from ineffective phrases to effective ones.

The improved hybrid optimizer algorithm, which tries to take the highest position in the search results for the effective phrases that can increase optimization efficiency by 45% compared to the classic algorithm.

4.5.5. Benefits for Advertising

Benefits of Artificial Intelligence for ad optimization:

- knows how to set bids for low-frequency phrases and phrases without conversions

- takes into account the associated conversions from GoogleAds, when setting bids (more data - more precisely a bid is set)

- can read the labels of the third-party systems (for example, Analytics).

5. Prospects for the use of Artificial Intelligence in healthcare

5.1. Personalized medicine and Deep Learning

Personalized medicine is based on the data related to the patient's condition, his/her medical history, the results of the functional studies and the information about treatment measures, the aforementioned device can assess the severity of the condition (extremely severe, moderate, etc.) or the degree of the disease. Thus, this will be followed by a proposed therapy based on all of the above facts. As a result, ML can rely on an existing database and factors such as blood pressure, age, weight, comorbidities (very often the presence of obesity, diabetes in patients with musculoskeletal diseases), and it can select the correct therapy in detail. In this case, forecasting is also used, since in this case its task is to choose the most optimal treatment strategy; predicting the development of the disease, its duration and outcome.

An example of the use of Artificial Intelligence in personalized medicine to predict the development of cancer and selection of the best treatment for each specific case is TreatmentMAP™, which was developed by MolecularHealth. TreatmentMAP™ compares patient-specific tumor genome information with the biomedical knowledge available worldwide and provides comprehensive molecular profiling of the cancer genome as a basis for subsequent analysis and the prescription of individual therapy options.[1]

TreatmentMAP™ provides the clinician with a reliable basis for making decisions regarding the choice of a medical drug for a particular patient.

TreatmentMAP™ helps physicians optimize treatment decisions for cancer patients with an advanced stage of the disease ,or when standard therapy has been depleted. This product provides

---

[1] The data from Presentation: Engineering the Medical Revolution. Precision Medicine in Germany (Molecular Health GmbH, 2015) were kindly given by Molecular Health Gmbh.

complete information regarding licensing and development of the status of investigational medicinal products as well as the available medicinal products in the market. TreatmentMAP™ also analyzes information from the clinical trials that match the molecular profile of each individual patient and analyzes risk factors for safe drug use.

In order to ensure the safety and further development of the medical value, TreatmentMAP ™ constantly verifies and updates databases in collaboration with world renowned cancer centers. The advantage of the TreatmentMAP ™ assay is that all known biomarkers can be analyzed and evaluated simultaneously. In comparison to the tests of a single gene, the physician receives much deeper informational content, since the individual complexity of the tumor is presented and gene interactions are identified. Moreover, there is no need to carry out several separate tests one at a time, which saves time and material. TreatmentMap ™ is the first registered medical product of this type in Europe for the personalized cancer medicine.[2] Molecular Health operates in Germany. The TreatmentMap™ tests are carried out at many laboratories in Germany.

TreatmentMap™ uses deep learning. In comparison to other products with similar purposes, a tumor analysis is performed by

---

[2] The data from the brochure: FAQs für EU. TreatmentMAP™. Für Ärzte und Patienten, Molecular Health GmbH were kindly given by Molecular Health Gmbh.

using the entire human genome, where all data that can be found in PubMed is used, and this includes all currently known clinical studies, all clinical trial records and all known drugs (23 million publications, 10,000 clinical studies, 22,000 medicines for the treatment of oncological diseases), as well as the holistic information about the patient (information on concomitant diseases and the interaction of drugs used by him/her). This allows very accurate prediction of the optimal treatment option with information on toxicity and about interaction of the pharmaceutical drugs[3]

5.2. An automated treatment plan and simulation of the preoperative planning stage

Clinical practices are increasingly incorporating automation systems, based on the analysis of existing databases and patient information. In the presence of certain symptoms, the system itself gives recommendations on methods of treatment, taking medications, etc., without taking the doctor's time to write such recommendations (cf. Langkafel 2014, loc.646-691).

In addition, AI is able to solve design and computational problems of any level and it can simulate, for example, optimal designs in orthopedics, research processes or create prototyping. The technology makes it possible to simulate the internal organs in

---

[3] The data from Presentation: Engineering the Medical Revolution. Precision Medicine in Germany (Molecular Health GmbH, 2015) were kindly given by Molecular Health Gmbh.

preparation for operations, preliminary study of implanted parts, etc. The exact size and shape of a defect in a particular bone is determined by a computed tomography. Physical 3D models are irreplaceable helpers to improve the quality of the surgical treatment and prosthetics (cf. Volosnikov 2013, p. n/a).

5.3. Robotization

The use of AI in the medical robotics has already gone beyond the DaVinchi controlled robot. Currently, robotics are controlled by a human doctor, but its use guarantees greater accuracy.

6. Orthopedic Clinic: set of processes using Artificial Intelligence in the framework of the medical institution

The orthopedic clinic is located in Moscow, Russia. It should be understood that in healthcare in Russia there is an exceptionally low level of implementation and use of technology based on AI e. According to the Russian Association of Developers and Users of Artificial Intelligence in Medicine "National Medical Knowledge Base", there are now about four thousand solutions in the field of AI in healthcare in the world. In Russia, if we now begin to recall all the proposals in this area, which are not even solutions, we will not be able to recall more than twenty (cf. Mekhanik 2020, p. n/a).

A significant difference between Russian medicine and medicine in Organisation for Economic Co-operation and Development (OECD) countries is its industrial backwardness, i.e., an extremely limited systematic approach to organizing work processes, setting measurable quality goals, economic justification, goal management and informatization (cf. Morozov 2018, p. n/a).

The Russian system of healthcare can be described as being in a state of crisis. Health indicators are deteriorating. The problems of accessibility and quality of care are becoming more acute. The unfortunate state of this sphere is becoming a serious social problem.

On the one hand, there is the total commercialization of health care and, on the other hand, there is the fact it is the lagging behind in technological terms and the mindset of doctors, who remain conservative. The European Center for Orthopedics and Pain Therapy, which has been working on the Russian market for 4 years, has introduced innovations and the use of the most advanced German technologies for diagnosis and treatment of the orthopedic and neurological diseases, and it has done experiments to test and use techniques with AI in those areas that do not contradict the rather outdated guidelines of the Russian Health Monitoring Agency, which is the regulatory body in the healthcare sector of the Russian Federation.

The following legislative problems can be identified:

1. Software in medicine is not separated into a separate class of products, requiring a different approach than that needed for equipment and pharmaceuticals. Therefore, registration of any product is mandatory, and this means considerable financial and time costs (cf. Mekhanik 2020, p. n/a).

2. For developers - obtaining the right to use the databases needed for work with AI. The main objection here is medical confidentiality. Currently, according to Federal Law 152 (cf. Federal Law 2006), it is impossible to use even depersonalized data, since it is necessary to obtain the patient's consent. (cf. Mekhanik 2020, p. n/a).

Despite the existing difficulties, the Clinic uses a number of AI-based products and applications.

6.1. Description of existing processes using Artificial Intelligence

Organization: Center for Orthopedics and Pain Therapy is an outpatient clinic. The clinic is also currently involved in a scientific study on pay-for-performance in medicine. Here, it is possible to use AI to determine quality parameters and evaluate treatment outcomes. In order to achieve even higher quality of service and at the same time reduce costs, the implementation of AI might contribute to this strategy and avoid price increasing that would otherwise not have been possible in a development of focus strategy. In a clinic, the machine learning can be used in numerous ways. The application of AI in the clinic, specializing in orthopedics enables one to see different capabilities of AI.

The clinic uses a number of platforms and software products that employ Artificial Intelligence or elements of it to varying degrees.

1.   The diagnostics performed by AI are based on MRT images. No doctor is able to instantly process all the information for each patient, summarize a large number of other similar medical records and immediately have a clear result. Therefore, machine learning and Artificial Intelligence are becoming an indispensable tool. If the task can be clearly formulated, then a specialized product can be created for the needs of the orthopedic clinic. At the moment, there is enough reliable data for machine learning that has been validated for many years. Based on this information, AI can be trained to recognize images with minute details that might otherwise be missed by a doctor. In addition, there is a huge database of various proven signs (history, symptoms, etc.) that are used to make a differential diagnosis and determine its severity.

2.   The clinic uses DIERS computer diagnostics of the musculoskeletal system with an optical analysis of posture and gait. Based on the data obtained after the diagnosis, the program bases its data on the analysis of the patient databases according to

the parameters of the optical image. As a result, it issues a comparative analysis and gives the doctor a presumptive diagnosis (for example, when analyzing the degree of curvature in scoliosis, an indication of problem areas such as muscles and joints is given; and a comparison with the zones of the feet and possible systemic diseases is made).

In addition, using a correlation model describing the relationship between the curvature of the surface and the vertebral bodies, makes it possible to perform a spatial (three-dimensional) reconstruction of the shape of the spine and determine the rotation of the individual vertebrae, or the position of the pelvis.

3.   Using language programs and speech recognition programs. Due to the fact that the team which ensures the functioning of the company and the clinic is international and 3 languages are constantly used (German, English, Russian), such as Google Translator and DeepL.

In addition, the clinic serves patients with Allianz international insurance. Many of these patients do not speak Russian, so speech recognition programs are used to better communicate with them.

4.   Artificial Intelligence in business processes. The clinic pays great attention to the optimization of all marketing processes. Amo CRM is used, which is integrated with the site, which includes various advertising channels, chat, and callback. In order to maintain patient records, and issue medical reports, the

clinic uses the Medesk program. These programs, although they do not use AI, are the basis for creating a database, which can be used to analyze work efficiency. Also, the call center uses a chat bot capable of answering the simplest questions to the patients and redistributing more complex requests to the call center's operators.

For example, before the introduction of automatization, the requesting process looked like this:

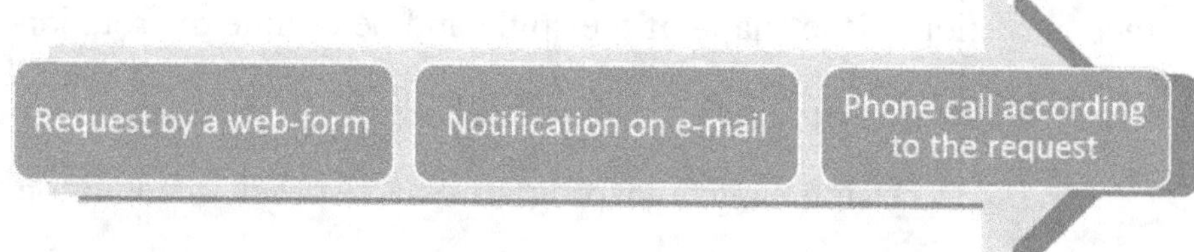

Figure 5. The process of processing applications before automatization.
(Own illustration)

There was a high probability of losing orders even at the entrance. Also, there was no control of processing and subsequent control over the arrival of the patient at the clinic. After the introduction of automation, a chatbot and the integration of several platforms with the CRM and the website, the process of a request for an appointment took the following form:

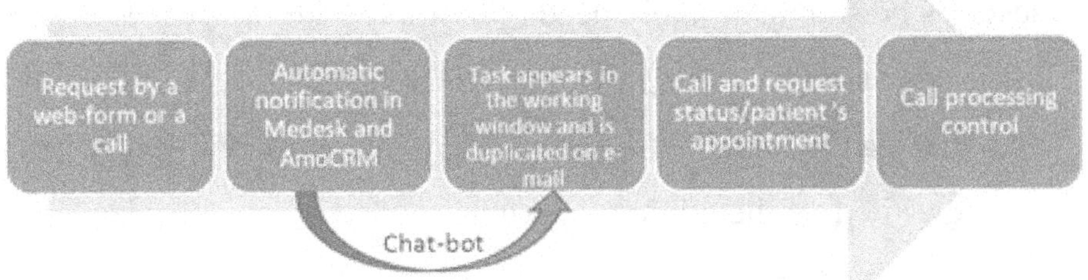

Figure 6. Application processing after automatzation

(Own illustration)

When integration and automatization are implemented, even at the initial stage, an Artificial Intelligence technology is applied, namely a chatbot. Thus, thanks to the automatization of the process to receive and process an application, a control appears along the entire chain - from the receipt of an application to its finalization. As a result, not only written requests are automatically entered into the database, but also requests from the site, and calls that come through the call-tracking Roistat.

According to the clinic data, thanks to automatization, it was possible to increase patient flow by 2.5 times.

6.2. Artificial Intelligence in marketing and advertising

During the development of the clinic, various Artificial Intelligence tools were introduced to optimize marketing. Thus, for example, there is a system of recommendations for services on the clinic's website. The user is shown an advertisement about the services he/she most likely needs. In order to do this, we focus on the user's reaction to the previous recommendations about services and the user's metadata: age, gender, and previous pages that he/she visited on the clinic's website.

Let's say that when a user, a 45-years-old man,has looked at the articles about back and lower back pain on the clinic's website, it is logical to assume that he has a backache and he needs manual therapy or a visit to an orthopedist. In order to automate the process of issuing such targeted recommendations, neural networks are used. They are quite complex, so we will look at a simple example based on the TensorRec library for Python:

First, we import needed libraries:

```
import numpy as np
import tensorrec
```

Then, as we assume we have data for user features, item features, and interactions (which is essentially feedback from the person about ads), we can build the model with default parameters and train it with this data.

```
model = tensorrec.TensorRec( )
model.fit(interactions, user_features,
item_features, epochs=10, verbose=True)
```

Now we have a trained model, so we can make predictions for all of the ads and all of the users we have.

```
preds =
model.predict(item_features=item_features,

            user_features=user_features)
```

Thus, using a simple Python algorithm, makes it possible to introduce a suitable recommendation system on the site.

The clinic advertising system uses various keywords, and one needs to understand on which words to focus on at any given time in order to maximize the flow of potential customers to the site, while reducing advertising costs or at least not increasing them. In order to do this, one can use a time series forecasting system (for example, ARIMA) and see how the growth in popularity of specific keywords depends on the time of day, weather, political situation, day of the week or month in the year. Understanding such dependencies can allow building an Artificial Intelligence bot that will remotely manage advertising campaigns to make advertising as effective as possible. The clinic can also use AI, that predicts the growth in popularity of specific keywords in real time and directs the budget towards them. At this stage, the clinic is collaborating with a Python programmer and collecting data to create its own algorithm.

At this stage, due to the insufficient amount of data so far, the algorithm is imperfect, but it helps to understand how to evaluate the budget for each type of ad.

Three months ago, the clinic switched to advertising its services using Origami. According to the first results, the Clinic's marketers noted an increase of circa 12% in applications received from advertising with an unchanged advertising budget. It is difficult to give a comparative description of the previous position and the present one with Origami, since the transition occurred at the time of the COVID-19 pandemic, which imposed a number of restrictions, including having a negative impact on the flow of patients to the clinic.

6.3. Prospects for Improving Healthcare
Processes by using Artificial Intelligence

The clinic's goal is leadership through cost savings. This strategy gives it the advantage of being profitable even in a highly competitive environment.

From the perspective of this strategy, the use of technologies based on Artificial Intelligence makes it possible to save on expensive labor of doctors and rehab specialists, as well as improve the work of the call center and save on advertising by optimizing campaigns using AI. This frees up physicians' time to advise and manage patients, and AI controlls processes associated with the routine procedures (such as physical therapy or rehabilitation exercises and procedures).

The use of robotics is also possible: a specialized robot-rehabilitation therapist. However, this machine requires heavy investment and at the moment such an investment is considered unprofitable by the clinic's management.

Another differentiation strategy is also in place, since the use of the latest technologies is not only a unique selling proposition, but also gives special prestige to the clinic. This strategy allows to offer consumers (patients) a unique method of service and market the product a unique, since at this stage such technologies are used extremely rarely in Russian clinics.

When introducing Artificial Intelligence into various processes at the clinic, it is necessary, first of all, to develop a holistic strategy.

This process should involve a cross-functional team with a clear understanding of the business program and goals. IT experts and specialists in the construction and methodology of all processes and areas of activity should participate here. It is extremely important to train doctors, since they will directly interact and to a large extent control the processes with AI or its elements.

AI in the work of a clinic is, first of all, a new technology, and any technology requires monitoring, technical support, and coordination with all software products of the company // clinic. These are the processes that the IT specialists and specially trained managers should manage.

6.4. Artificial Intelligence implementation challenges

The problems, associated with the implementation of Artificial Intelligence can be divided into 3 groups: technical, economic and psychological.

- Cost-effectiveness of using Artificial Intelligence in medicine: the introduction of AI has high costs: machinery, equipment, implementation period (for example, the aforementioned advertisement requires a long period for adjustments), staff training, etc.

- Ethical issues: the most sensitive area is obtaining the right to use databases that are needed for AI learning. In fact, the very concept of "intelligence" is very conditional here, we are talking about neural networks, i.e., conditionally unsupervised systems that need sets of labeled data for learning, similar to how children need pictures with objects when they learn to speak and generally learn concepts. In order to teach a neural network to recognize lung cancer, it needs to view a large number of such images, and they need to be taken from patients. The main objection is medical confidentiality: now all our data will be stolen and something will be found out. However, firstly, we are not talking about personal data - no one needs it. AI learning needs depersonalized, impersonal data. However, even here there are problems that block its use. Because there is a danger of identifying the patient under certain conditions, even from depersonalized data.

Other problems of ethical nature are bias, relations between robots (machines) and people, where the question is raised in a reciprocal way: how people behave towards machines (robot rights) and how machines are a threat to humanity (singularity).

• Technical problems (lack of data, verification): the need for powerful computers to process large amounts of data (especially when it comes to image processing) in adequate time intervals.

• Psychological and socio-cultural factors. Fears constantly arise: what if we are doing something wrong there? (cf. Mekhanik 2020, p. n/a)

Below, some of the problems associated with introducing AI into everyday life in general and into medicine in particular are discussed in more details:

6.4.1. Invasion of Privacy

The problem of data is much broader than the question of using it for AI. It is also a separate issue for personal medicine. If one wants to have a personalized approach to treatment, then he or she must enable the doctor who will provide a person with this service to collect one's data from different sources, down to what one buys in the store, what and how one eats, what is the quality of water where one lives, and so on. We are talking about the need to analyze multimodal data about a person, about the need to compare data from various sources about his/her life and behavior, about the need to analyze the lifestyle of each person. Thus, it turns out that even if one erases his/her surname from his/her data, then it will still be easy to estimate one's surname using all these tags.

Protection of data and personal information in the medical field is a very sensitive topic from the point of view of legislators as it concerns highly personal information. If we use AI even in a call center, we need to protect information (especially personal data and diagnoses) from leaks and misuse (cf. Bohr/Memarzadeh 2020, pp.494-496).

6.4.2. Can Artificial Intelligence be trusted?

There is a question: to what extent can AI be trusted in making diagnoses, because all medicine is based on the principle - "do not harm". If AI makes a diagnosis, for example, any imperfections in the MRT images (for example, a dot) can change the whole diagnosis.

Some researchers argue that, due to small errors in the input data, a completely wrong diagnosis can be made at the output.

For example, in image recognition, some details (for example, a tumor) may be missed or, on the contrary, added. The slightest distortion in the image, which can be caused by a simple movement of the patient, greatly degrades the results of image recognition (cf. Antun et al. 2020, p. n/a).

6.4.3. Loss of Human Jobs

There is no doubt that AI is able to process huge amounts of information and issue solutions based on this analysis in a very short time. What normally would take years, a machine can do in a matter of minutes. According to the McKinsey Global Institute report around 800 million jobs could be lost worldwide because of automation by 2030 (cf. Manyika et al. 2017, p. n/a). Consequently, not only an economic conflict is arising, but also a social one.

6.4.4. Overfitting and Underfitting.

Overfitting and Underfitting are significant machine learning problems.

In machine learning, overfitting is a phenomenon when one constructs a training, and algorithm is obtained that works too well for the examples that participated in the training (i.e., examples from a training sample), but does not work well enough for the examples that did not participate in the training (i.e. examples from the test sample). This is due to the fact that when constructing such an algorithm in the training sample, some random patterns are found that are absent in the general population.

Underfitting is another phenomenon in machine learning where the complexity of the model prevents it from learning complex trends in the dataset (cf. Aich 2019, p. n/a).

6.4.5. Artificial Intelligence Bias. Variance. Black box.

Bias is used to allow a machine learning model to learn in a simplified way and it is injected into the model in order to achieve the simplest possible model. Simplification can result in a bias that, in turn, can lead to oversimplification of the model and, therefore, to its unreliability (cf. Aich 2019, p. n/a). Bias models tend to be underfitting, the model is not being trained and having low accuracy. The bias model is simply not capable of solving more complex problems.

Artificial Intelligence is created by human, and people are sometimes very biased towards various areas of society: gender, religion, nationality, race, political views - all this can be a point of conflict in the human world. This same bias is carried over to the world of machines and technology (cf. Bohr/Memarzadeh 2020, pp. 493-494). In addition, AI can fail in algorithms due to errors in the data, which it has been trained on. For example, IBM Watson has partnered with Dr. Anderson's Texas Cancer Center to identify and treat cancer in patients. However, due to incorrect data submitted to the system, this system has failed, as it gave completely incorrect medical recommendations to patients. Currently, the only way to overcome bias is to manually correct the bias in the development and training of AI systems, as well as on the stage of selection and preparation of data (cf. Bohr/Memarzadeh 2020, p. 491).

Another problem related to Artificial Intelligence training is variance. It appears when the model works well on the trained dataset, but does not work well with a dataset which it has not been trained on (cf. Aich 2019, p. n/a). A high variance model will tend to be overly complex. This leads to overfitting. A model with a high variance will have a very high training accuracy, but it will have a low testing accuracy.

Bias and variance are two different problems with AI, but they are interrelated at the same time: "if the bias of a model is decreased, the variance of the model automatically increases" (Aich 2019, p. n/a) . Almost any model has one or another deviation, as a result of which the so-called Bias-Variance Tradeoff.

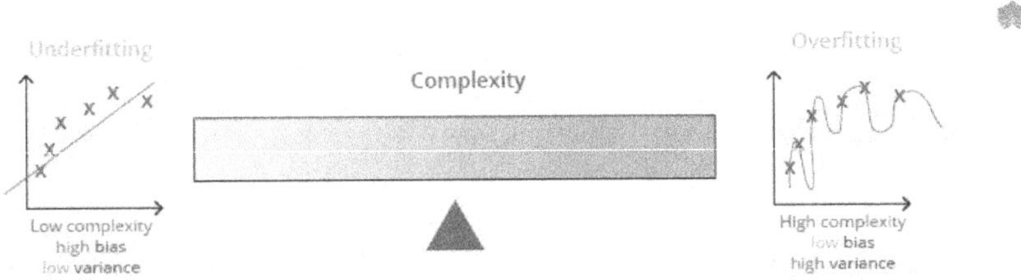

Figure 7. Bias-variance Tradeoff Graph. (Aich 2019)

Black box is one of the reasons why bias is so prevalent in machine learning. Many types of machine learning algorithms, especially unsupervised algorithms, work opaquely, or as a black box for the developer. Many models are untraceable to data scientists, and it remains unexplained why they produce a particular result. This makes it extremely difficult to identify cases of bias or other model failures (cf. Bohr/Memarzadeh 2020, pp. 493-494).

The logic behind these conclusions is incomprehensible and this leads to uncertainty about the correctness of the achieved results. How AI came to a particular conclusion is an essential information that is important for drawing up a treatment plan.

6.4.6. Robot-Human Relations: Robot Rights

Spielberg's fiction movie A.I. (Artificial Intelligence) is about such problems in the aspect of science fiction, but these relationships are becoming more real every day. In this regard, the attention of many researchers, scientists and entrepreneurs has been directed toward technological singularity. This is a hypothetical moment when, according to the supporters of this concept, technological progress will become so rapid and complex that it will be beyond the reach of human understanding.

Singularity is the moment in time when computers in all their incarnations will become smarter than humans. When this happens, computers will be able to grow exponentially compared to themselves and reproduce themselves, and their intelligence will be billions of times faster than the human intelligence. According to the forecasts, this moment may come within 10 years, namely in 2030. The main proponent of this idea is Raymond Kurzweil, who believes that the thirties of this century will be marked by such a level of development in Artificial (non-biological) Intelligence, that will demand to recognize the fact that it is conscious. From this moment on, the border between human and artificial consciousness begins to blur (cf. Kurzweil 2005, p.35). This idea is supported by Elon Musk, who believes that AI is a direct threat to humanity (cf. Cuthbertson 2020, p. n/a). However, not all scientists support this concept, asserting that thechnological development occurs along the S-curve, and at the end of the last century, a slowdown in its acceleration began.

Economic impacts of using Artificial Intelligence as seen with the example of an orthopedic clinic.

7.1. Survey

In order to establish an involvement of the clinic employees in the process of introducing Artificial Intelligence in their work and to acquire their opinion on the benefits of using AI in the clinic's activities from the point of view of the new reality of our time, a survey was conducted.

The clinic staff was asked to answer 10 questions of the questionnaire via google.forms:

1. Do you think that Artificial Intelligence technologies are useful to humans?

2. Do you think that the introduction of technologies with Artificial Intelligence will help in your work?

3. Have you used Artificial Intelligence technologies in your work or in another area? If so, please specify where exactly.

4. Do you think that the introduction of Artificial Intelligence can negatively affect you?

5. Do you think that Artificial Intelligence cannot fully perform your work and that humans do better?

6. Name the areas of the clinic in which the Artificial Intelligence can be effective

7. Name the benefits that Artificial Intelligence can have in the work of the clinic

8. What is the obstacle to the wider use of Artificial Intelligence in the clinic?

- Personal data law

- Patients' distrust // staff's distrust

- Technical difficulties

- Low information technological literacy

-       Insufficient data for Artificial Intelligence

-       Other

9. What do you think? Is the introduction of technologies with Artificial Intelligence economically profitable for the clinic?

10. Do you think that Artificial Intelligence will become a threat to humanity in the future?

7.2. Survey Results

The survey involved 19 employees of the clinic (Total number of the clinic staff is 21 persons, so 90,48% of staff participated in the survey, incl. 8 (42,1%) – physicians, 3 (15,8%) managers, 3 (15,8%) administrators, 2 (10,5%) IT department staff, 2 (10,5%) SMM managers, 1 (5,3%) translator.

Question (1): 100% of respondents answered with Yes. As a result, we can conclude that no one questions the benefits of using the technologies with Artificial Intelligence.

Question (2): 15,8% of employees believe that AI does not help in their work. Moreover, all those who answered negatively are doctors.

Question (3): 26,3% of respondents note that they have never used AI before. However, this question is, rather, more indicative of a lack of understanding in which applications and programs this technology is used. Prediction is used in navigation, which is used by absolutely everyone in Moscow, and in the weather forecast, and in other similar programs on a daily basis, where most do not even think that this is an Artificial Intelligence technology. The remaining 66.7% note the following areas with the use of products with elements of AI:

- Marketing and Advertising (Origami);
- Applications for translation, incl. google translator and deepl;
- Applications for speech recognition;
- Search algorithms;
- Using AI when building reports;
- Auto navigation (*for drivers);
- Buoy and ADA applications for diagnostics;
- Chat bots.

Moreover, most often one has encountered AI in marketing and advertising, in the process of communication with banks, in everyday life - when using navigation programs and an online translator.

<u>Question (4)</u>: Concerning whether or not the introduction of AI can negatively affect you, 68,4% do not see a threat, but the other 31,6% believe that the use of Artificial Intelligence can lead to a reduction in their workplace. In this case, it is interesting to note that none of the doctors notes a threat from AI. Mainly,

administration employees see a threat to their job, where chatbot technology, which is rapidly gaining popularity, can be used.

Question (5): 84,2% of respondents believe that AI is not capable of fully performing their work, and a human can do better. The employees who answered this question in a negative manner are managers and an administrators who work with advertising and with CRM.

Question (6): For the clinic, the respondents noted that the following areas could see the effective use of AI:

- surgery, standard operations;

- remote diagnostics;

- diagnostics of the musculoskeletal system using the DIERS equipment;

- robot assistant (cleaning, disinfection);

- diagnosis and treatment plan;

- call center: chatbots, messaging, patient registration, tracking records;

- electronic patient record;

- advertising and marketing strategies.

Question (7): employees note the following areas where AI can be effective:

- Increasing the number of patients through the use of Artificial Intelligence in advertising;

-        Improving the quality of services and speed of work, saving time;

-        Fast diagnosis for effective early ctreatment;

-        Quick selection of treatment and medication;

-        Easing pressure on the staff and the budget of the clinic, since AI is cheaper than human labor;

-        Automation of processes and reduction of human errors;

-        Simplification of the work of administrators, accuracy;

-        Performing routine work instead of people, thereby increasing the creativity of employees;

-        Reducing the advertising budget with an increase in the number of patients.

In general, the emphasis is on speed, quality and the processes' optimization.

<u>Question (8)</u>: it is possible to choose several answer options about obstacles to the introduction of AI into the activities of the clinic, the leading negative factor noted was distrust on the part of patients (78,9%) and technical difficulties (73,7%). The third most important factor is was compliance with the Personal Data Law (36,8%). This problem is especially severe for doctors and administrators who work directly with patients.

Question (9): 78,9% of respondents consider the introduction of Artificial Intelligence technologies to be cost-effective for the operation of the clinic. In terms of benefits,the following was noted:

- Reduction and optimization of marketing costs; advertising works better;
- Increasing in the number of patients through the optimization and automation of request processing;
- Artificial Intelligence works 24/7 in an automated mode;
- Increasing the speed of processing patient documentation (for doctors);
- Reduction of staff, reduction of personnel costs.

As a disadvantage, it is noted that the introduction of AI requires heavy investments and a considerable amount of resources, and jobs are lost.

Question (10): it was asked as an additional one in order to understand the attitude of the clinic staff toward singularity and the ethical issues of using AI.

36,8% of those surveyed do not see a threat to humanity in the future, but the majority (47,4%) are of opinion that AI will become a real threat to humanity. In addition, respondents note that the threat does not come directly from AI (5,3%), but from the person behind it. They (5,3%) also see a threat in job cuts and assume that there will be a certain symbiosis between AI and humans (5,3%), since AI will not be able to perform work as efficiently as humans do.

This survey demonstrates the situation with AI implementation in the clinic and human life, and confirms the trends, problems and prospects discussed above.

8. Final Conclusion

AI is one of the most promising factors for the health care development, both from the point of view of medicine itself in various areas - diagnostics, telemedicine and chatbots, personalized medicine, robotization - and in the field of management of a medical institucion and marketing strategies.

Based on the aforementioned facts, we can draw the following conclusions about the prospects for introducing AI into the activities of a medical organization.

8.1 Advantages

1.   The effectiveness of the activities of professional healthcare providers will increase. Thanks to the use of Artificial Intelligence in a medical practice, the time for making a diagnosis is reduced, while the accuracy of the diagnosis and the effectiveness of treatment is increased. Doctors can spend more

time on prevention, monitoring compliance, or new patients. The quality of treatment and the involvement of patients in the treatment process is increased by reducing the amount of time spent. In other words, the physician avoids trial and error. Artificial Intelligence may have a major role in this: it can be used to make a more accurate diagnosis. This technology is already being used in medicine, so its introduction to an orthopedic clinic is quite possible and could significantly reduce the costs of both the clinic and the patients who attend it, as there werewould be no costs for unnecessary consultations, tests, etc. and the choice of treatment scheme would be optimized. Such use of AI would certainly bring new value to the clinic. Moreover, AI will reduce the time, required to the proper medical treatment, and – most of all - it will save the patients' time. As a result of the introduction of AI in a clinic environment, the patients will have an access to high-tech treatment and be able to get a quick and accurate diagnosis, followed by adequate and optimal treatment program. Doctors will have in their hands a tool for a quick and an accurate diagnosis by using Artificial Intelligence (prediction) and the medical treatment selection (judgment). The doctor executes this treatment program (action) by using some elements of robotics (action).

2.   A reduction of costs for the patients (when the patient pays for the treatment) or the health care system as a whole (when the state pays for treatment) can be achieved while improving the

health of a given patient. The introduction of AI aims to help the patient improve his/her condition or cure the disease more quickly while placing primary emphasis or preventing the chronic course of the disease. The patient is not prescribed unnecessary, additional, often unnecessary tests and analyzes, which significantly reduces the cost of treatment. As a result, the patient needs fewer visits to the doctor, or communication with the doctor turns into a virtual space. Lower costs for drugs and medical / laboratory research are needed both in the short term and in the long term. In addition, with the help of AI programs, it is possible to create incentives and controls for the patient to precisely follow the recommendations of the attending physician.

3.   Artificial Intelligence can be used to operate a call center and track the company's reputation, which will reduce the cost of attracting and training new personnel, since the existing workforce is able to fully and quickly process incoming requests by using AI.

4.   The use of the Artificial Intelligence-based program Origami resulted in a reduction in advertising costs and an increase in the number of applications / patient flow. In addition, the volume of work for marketers was reduced, which made it possible to develop other areas of attracting patients to the clinic (for example, interaction with partners, making contracts with insurance companies, more intensive work in social networks).

5.   Reasonable and thoughtful implementation as well as the use of AI can reduce personnel costs. Thus, for example, with the help of applications based on AI, one can improve the work of the HR department to attract new professionals to the industry or use AI to free up the employees' time, as well.

8.2. Disadvantages

1.   Insufficient level of technical equipment in the clinic. Many Artificial Intelligence-based applications require powerful computer hardware. This is especially true for applications that analyze images, which is the main goal of the orthopedic clinic, where the analysis of MRI images is necessary. Equipping a small clinic with this equipment can be an unjustified investment that will not have a return on investment and it will not pay off.

2.   Rather weak computer literacy of staff. Work with almost all applications requires good computer and technical literacy among the staff, which is not always a given. Personnel training requires high financial costs. For this reason, the issue of staff retention in the workplace is of great importance, since it is difficult for new employees to start a full-fledged work process without expensive training.

3.   For the management, an introduction of AI into the processes of the clinic makes it necessary to take into account the established tasks in each specific case. In a small clinic, it is important to have a clear understanding of how much cost and

speed, as well as the ability to adapt its functionality for a specific task will be necessary before technologies or robotics with AI are introduced. Having simple control is important so that the clinic staff can independently use all the functionality of the introduced Artificial Intelligence in use there, which depends on the task at hand. Reliability and usability are also important. A clear assessment is needed of how the benefits will commensurate with the cost of implementation.

***

Artificial Intelligence is developing now with amazing speed. Artificial intelligence is closely linked to the concept of scientific and technological progress. Despite the fact that AI is still far from being perfect, the improvement of its algorithms is happening every day, and in the near future AI will enter our daily lives even more widely and will become an indispensable tool in healthcare.

References

Agadzhanov, M. (2015): IBM Watson for Oncology: pomoshch'
kognitivnoy sistemy v bor'be s rakom [Agadzhanov, M. (2015): IBM
Watson for Oncology: helping the cognitive   system fight cancer],
http://www.interface.ru/home.asp?artId=37935 [05.07.2020].

Aich, A. (2019): What is Bias-Variance Tradeoff in Machine Learning,
https://www.knowledgehut.com/blog/data-science/bias-variance-
tradeoff-in-machine-   learning [12.07.2020].

Antun, V./Renna, F./Poon, C./Adcock, B./Hansen, A. C. (2020): On
instabilities of deep   learning in image reconstruction and the
potential costs of AI ,
https://www.pnas.org/content/early/2020/05/08/1907377117
[18.07.2020].

Arrieta, A. B./Díaz-Rodríguez, N./Del Ser, J./Bennetot, A./Tabik,
S./Barbado, A./Garcia,   S./Gil-Lopez, S./Molina, D./Benjamins,
R./Chatila, R./Herrera, F. (2020): Explainable
Artificial Intelligence (XAI): Concepts, taxonomies, opportunities and
challenges toward   responsible AI,
https://www.sciencedirect.com/science/article/pii/S1566253519308103
3   [22.07.2020].

Banzhaf, W./Goodman, E./Sheneman, L./Trujillo, L./Worzel,
B. (2020): Genetic   Programming Theory and
Practice XVII, Switzerland: Springer Nature.

Barr, A./Feigenbaum, E. A. (1981): The Handbook of Artificial
Intelligence, Volume 1, Los   Altos, CA: William Kaufmann,
Inc.

Berners-Lee, T./Shadbolt, N. (2011): There's gold to be mined from all our
data. The Times,
http://www.thetimes.co.uk/tto/opinion/columnists/article3272618.ece
[29.06.2020].

Bohr, A./Memarzadeh, K. (eds.) (2020): Artificial Intelligence in
Healthcare, London: Elsevier Inc.

Chen, J. (2020): Neural Network Definition,
        https://www.investopedia.com/terms/n/neuralnetwork.asp
        [29.06.2020].

Copeland, B.J. (2020): Artificial intelligence,
        https://www.britannica.com/technology/artificial-intelligence
        [14.08.2020].

Cuthbertson, A. (2020): Elon Musk claims AI will overtake humans 'in less
        than five years',   https://www.independent.co.uk/life-style/gadgets-
        and-tech/news/elon-musk-artificial-   intelligence-ai-singularity-
        a9640196.html [01.08.2020].

Dacombe, J. (2017): An introduction to Artificial Neural Networks (with
        example),   https://medium.com/@jamesdacombe/an-introduction-to-
        artificial-neural-networks-with-   example-ad459bb6941b
        [15.07.2020]

Dasgupta, N. (2018): Practical Big Data Analytics, Birmingham: Packt
        Publishing Ltd.

De, S. (2017): Healthcare artificial intelligence market to record a
        commendable CAGR of   40% over 2017-2024, U.S. to
        prominently drive the regional growth,
        https://www.fractovia.org/news/industry-research-report/healthcare-
        artificial-intelligence-   market [15.07.2020].

Fedak, V. (2018): Top 10 Most Popular AI Models,
        https://dzone.com/articles/top-10-most-popular-ai-models
        [05.07.2020].

Federal Law of 27.07.2006 N152-FZ "On Personal Data"
        https://pd.rkn.gov.ru/authority/p146/p164/ [21.07.2020].

Groves, P./Kayyali, B./Knott, D./Van Kuiken, S. (2013): The Big Data
        revolution in Health-   care – Accelerating value and innovation,
        McKinsey&Company – Center for US Health   System Reform
        Business Technology Office,
        https://www.mckinsey.com/industries/healthcare-systems-and-

services/our-insights/the-big-   data-revolution-in-us-health-care#
[03.07.2020].

Gusev, A.V./Dobridnyuk, S.L. (2017) Iskusstvennyy intellekt v meditsine: i
zdravookhranenii, v: Informatsionnoye obshchestvo [Gusev,
A.V./Dobridnyuk, S.L. (2017): Artificial Intelligence in Medicine
and Healthcare, in: Information Society], № 4-5, pp. 78-93.

Hernandez, D. (2019): Computers Can Now Bluff Like a Poker Champ.
Better, Actually, https://www.wsj.com/articles/computers-can-
now-bluff-like-a-poker-champ-better-actually- 11562873541
[04.08.2020].

Hoffman, A. (2016): What is the difference between all the
companies working on machine learning?,
https://www.quora.com/What-is-the-difference-between-all-the-
companies-working-on- machine-learning [13.07.2020].

Joshi, K./Sumant, O. (2020): AI in Healthcare Market by Offering
(Hardware, Software, and Services), Algorithm (Deep Learning,
Querying Method, Natural Language Processing, and Context
Aware Processing) Application (Robot-Assisted Surgery, Virtual
Nursing Assistant, Administrative Workflow Assistance, Fraud
Detection, Dosage Error Reduction, Clinical Trial Participant
Identifier, Preliminary Diagnosis, and Others), and End user
(Healthcare Providers, Pharmaceutical & Biotechnology
Companies, Patients, and Payer): Global Opportunity Analysis
and Industry Forecast, 2019-2027,
https://www.alliedmarketresearch.com/artificial-intelligence-in-
healthcare-market [21.07.2020].

Kirk, J. (2017): TensorRec: A Recommendation Engine Framework in
TensorFlow, https://hackernoon.com/tensorrec-a-
recommendation-engine-framework-in-tensorflow- d85e4f0874e8
[28.07.2020].

Kurzweil, R. (2005): The Singularity Is Near: When Humans Transcend
Biology, New York: Viking Press.

Kuznetzov, M. (2018): Meditsina budushchego — eto tselaya
        ekosistema [Kuznetzov, M.   (2018): Medicine of the future -
        it's an entire ecosystem],
        http://health.rbc.ru/articles/treatment/medicina-budushego-
        eto-celaya-ekosistema/ /   [04.07.2020].

Langkafel, P. (2014): Big Data in Medizin und Gesundheitswirtschaft:
        Diagnose, Therapie,   Nebenwirkungen, Heidelberg: Medhochzwei
        Verlag GmbH.

Lee, J. H./Shin, J./Realff, M. J. (2018): Machine learning: Overview
        of the recent progresses   and implications for the process
        systems engineering field, in: Computers & Chemical
        Engineering, Vol. 114, pp. 111-121.

Manyika, J./Lund, S./Chui, M./ Bughin, J./Woetzel, J./Batra, P./Ko,
        R./Sanghvi, S. (2017):   Jobs lost, jobs gained: Workforce
        transitions in a time of automation,
        https://www.mckinsey.com/featured-insights/future-of-work/jobs-lost-
        jobs-gained-what-   the-future-of-work-will-mean-for-jobs-skills-and-
        wages [23.07.2020].

Mekhanik, A. (2020): Iskusstvennyy intellekt preodolevayet
        prepyatstviya [Mechanic, A.   (2020): Artificial Intelligence
        Overcomes Obstacles],
        https://expert.ru/2020/08/5/iskusstvennyij-intellekt-
        preodolevaet-prepyatstviya/   [12.08.2020]

Mitchell, J. (2017): BIDMC researchers use artificial intelligence to identify
        bacteria quickly and accurately, https://www.bidmc.org/about-
        bidmc/news/bidmc-researchers-use-artificial-intelligence-to-identify-
        bacteria-quickly-and-accurately [17.07.2020].

Monnappa, A. (2020): Data Science vs. Big Data vs. Data Analytics,
        https://www.simplilearn.com/data-science-vs-big-data-vs-data-
        analytics-article   [03.08.2020].

Morozov, S. (2018): Virtual'nyy doktor. Kak budet rabotat' iskusstvennyy
        intellekt v meditsine [Morozov, S .: Virtual Doctor. How artificial
        intelligence will work in medicine],

https://www.forbes.ru/tehnologii/356327-virtualnyy-doktor-kak-budet-
rabotat- iskusstvennyy-intellekt-v-medicine [24.07.2020].

Ng, A. (2016): What Artificial Intelligence Can and Can't Do Right Now,
https://hbr.org/2016/11/what-artificial-intelligence-can-and-cant-do-
right-now [16.07.2020]

Nunez, A. (2017): New Startup Claims Its AI-Powered Chatbot Can
Diagnose Illness Better Than Any Doctor,
https://www.menshealth.com/health/a19543125/artificial-
intelligence-doctor-app/ [05.08.2020].

O'Neil, C. (2016): Weapons of math destruction, New York: Crown Publishing
Group.

Ostrovskiy, K. i kollektiv avtorov J'son & Partners Consulting (2017):
Iskusstvennyy intellekt (II) / Artificial Intelligence (AI) kak klyuchevoy
faktor tsifrovizatsii global'noy ekonomiki [Ostrovsky, K. and the team
of authors J'son & Partners Consulting (2017): Artificial Intelligence
(AI) as a Key Factor of the Global Economy's Digitalization],
https://json.tv/ict_telecom_analytics_view/iskusstvennyy-intellekt-ii-
artificial-intelligence- ai-kak-klyuchevoy-faktor-tsifrovizatsii-
globalnoy-ekonomiki-20170222045241 [19.07.2020]

Rival, S. (2018): AI in Marketing [Video]. YouTube. URL,
https://www.youtube.com/watch?v=FYMjXD3G
Y&lc=z23hgfkpdnfjyt0n1acdp431kuaxf khbz5py54gjhedw03c010c
[15.07. 2020]

Rosenfeld, A./Zemel, R. K. /Tsotsos, J. (2018): The Elephant in the Room,
https://arxiv.org/abs/1808.03305 [09.07.2020]

Ross, C./Swetlitz, I. (2017): IBM pitched its Watson supercomputer as a
revolution in cancer care. It's nowhere close,
https://www.statnews.com/2017/09/05/watson-ibm-cancer/
[28.07.2020].

Russel, S./Norvig, P. (2016): Artificial Intelligence. A Modern
Approach, 3th ed., Harlow: Pearson Education Ltd.

Shum, H. (2017): Microsoft Build 2017: Microsoft AI – Amplify human
	ingenuity, https://blogs.microsoft.com/blog/2017/05/10/microsoft-
	build-2017-microsoft-ai-amplify-	human-
	ingenuity/#sm.0000wf98mzy2dfiyr722jw [10.06.2020].

Smith, B./Linden, G. (2017): Two decades of recommender systems at
	amazon.com, in: IEEE Internet Computing, Vol. 21, Issue 3,
	https://doi.org/10.1109/MIC.2017.72
	[16.07.2020]

Stiedemann, A. (2020): Complete Architectural Details of all EfficientNet
	Models, https://morioh.com/p/ebb64276117e [03.08.2020]

Topol, E. (2019): Deep Medicine: How Artificial Intelligence Can
	Make Healthcare Human Again, New York: Basic Books.

Volosnikov, A. (2013): Vozmozhnosti vnedreniya sistem
	avtomatizirovannogo proyektirovaniya v klinicheskuyu
	praktiku meditsinskikh uchrezhdeniy travmatologii i
	ortopedii [Volosnikov, A. (2013): Possibilities to implement
	computer-aided design systems in the clinical practice of
	the medical institutions in the area of traumatology and
	orthopedics],https://sapr.ru/article/23814 [30.07.2020].

Wegert, T. (2016): A Robot Named Albert Wants to Revolutionize Digital
	Advertising, https://contently.com/2016/10/27/robot-albert-digital-
	advertising/ [29.07.2020].

www.ingramcontent.com/pod-product-compliance
Lightning Source LLC
Chambersburg PA
CBHW061249140726

47998CB00006B/2169